Inflammation

Anti-Inflammatory Diet

The Ultimate Guide on How to Overcome Inflammation Naturally Without Relying On Medication

Introduction

End inflammation naturally by implementing the natural strategies in this book.

Inflammation is one word that evokes thoughts of pain and aches. However, did you know that it is a sign that your body is actually fighting to heal?

Yes, when your body is injured, acute inflammation occurs. Your cells release chemicals, which leads to internal or external swelling. As a result, white blood cells are attracted to the inflamed area and they quickly begin to repair the damage. In other words, acute inflammation is good for you. It leads to healing.

However, another type of inflammation can be your greatest enemy.

This is chronic inflammation. This type of inflammation is the root cause of diseases such as rheumatoid arthritis, obesity, lupus, Alzheimer's disease, Parkinson's disease, heart disease, premature aging and cancer amongst others. It is bad news. It wreaks havoc on your immune system and robs you off the energy you need to enjoy your life.

Thanks to this book, you can do something about chronic inflammation. In this book, you will learn more about chronic inflammation, the symptoms and causes of inflammation, the anti-inflammatory diet and the various recipes you can use to heal your immune system and boost your energy.

I hope you enjoy it!

Table of Contents

Introduction 2

Chapter 1: The Anti-Inflammatory Diet Unmasked 7

Chapter 2: What Causes Inflammation ____ 10

Chapter 3: Diet And Inflammation _____ 14

The Benefits Of The Anti-Inflammatory Diet _____ 17

Chapter 4: Vegetables For Fighting Inflammation _____ 24

Chapter 5: Fruits That Fight Inflammation 28

Chapter 6: Drinks _____ 30

Chapter 7: Great Protein And Fats For Dealing With Inflammation _____ 33

   Proteins _____ 33
   Healthy Fats _____ 34

Chapter 8: Whole Grains That Can Address Inflammation _____ 37

Chapter 9: Herbs And Spices _____ 39

The Anti-Inflammatory Diet Recipes ____ 42

Breakfast Recipes _____ 42

Amaranth Porridge with Roasted Pears _____ 42
Whole 30 Sweet Potato Protein Breakfast Bowl 44
Turkey Apple Breakfast Hash (AIP) _____ 46
Maple-Baked Rice Porridge Recipe With Fruit_ 48

Lunch Recipes _____ 50

Deep Dish Falafel Pizza _____ 50
Sweet Potato 'Rice' Casserole _____ 53
Anti-Inflammatory Orange Chicken And Spinach Salad _____ 55
Curried Red Lentil And Swiss Chard Soup ____ 58
Anti-Inflammatory Salad _____ 60
White Turkey Chili And Avocado _____ 62
Chicken and Snap Pea Stir-Fry _____ 64
Smoked Salmon Salad With Green Goddess Dressing _____ 66
Black Bean With Creamy Cashew Dressing ____ 68
Puttanesca-Style Beans and Greens _____ 71
Orecchiette Pasta with Kale Pesto _____ 73
Loaded Sesame Ginger Salmon Salad _____ 75

Desserts, Appetizers And Snacks _____ 77

Low Carb Coconut Crunch _____ 77
Fried Plantains with Cinnamon _____ 79
1 ripe plantain, peeled _____ 79

Two Ingredient Pumpkin Ice Cream _____ 80

Homemade Pumpkin Applesauce _____ 81

3-Ingredient Banana Pudding Recipe _____ 83

Slow Cooker Applesauce (without sugar) _____ 84

Turmeric Broccoli Chicken Roll Ups _____ 85

The Two-Week Meal Plan Table (Sample) 87

Week 1 _____ 87

Week 2 _____ 88

Overcoming The Common Challenges, Fears And Uncertainties Concerning The Anti-Inflammatory Diet _____ 89

Enhance The Anti-Inflammatory Effects With Increased Physical Activity _____ 98

Conclusion _____ 102

Chapter 1: The Anti-Inflammatory Diet Unmasked

The anti-inflammatory diet has to do with eating certain foods that help counteract inflammation. In order to understand fully the importance of the anti-inflammatory diet, you first need to understand why you need it in the first place.

As already stated, there are two types of inflammation. The first one is acute inflammation that leads to healing and the second type is chronic inflammation. Chronic inflammation is basically unresolved acute inflammation. It doesn't go away quickly. It can last for weeks, months and in some cases, years.

Think of it this way. If you knock your knee on the door, the area swells but the swelling goes away in a day or two. This is an instance of acute inflammation. Once the damage is repaired, you go on with your life.

Now think of having a red, swollen area of your body that stays like that for weeks, months or years. Now imagine having many such parts due to your body being constantly bombarded with substances that cause inflammation. It's like your body is always in the fight mode. It is being over taxed.

As a result, it gets confused and starts attacking anything on its path including healthy body cells. This is chronic inflammation. It doesn't discriminate. It attacks healthy cells and causes various health issues.

What's more, you may not even recognize you suffer from chronic inflammation because it may not be accompanied by pain or external swelling. However, recognizing the various symptoms of inflammation is the first step to healing.

Symptoms of inflammation include:

- Redness
- Fatigue
- Swollen joints
- Joint pain
- Chronic pain
- Ulcers
- Diarrhea or constipation
- Irritable Bowel Syndrome (IBS)
- Water retention
- Acne
- Eczema
- Brain fog
- Headaches and migraines
- Heartburn
- Obesity

- Food cravings

- Fever

- Chills

- Swollen lymph nodes

As you can see, there are varied symptoms of inflammation. You may exhibit some and not others. However, the bottom line is, once your body is bombarded with inflammation, your immune system will be unable to effectively do its work of guarding you against disease. It will be compromised.

As such, you will be prone to all the diseased associated with chronic inflammation. This is why it is vital to keep chronic inflammation at bay. One thing that will help you do this is knowing the causes of inflammation. This knowledge will help you take steps to avoid or greatly minimize inflammation.

Chapter 2: What Causes Inflammation

Inflammation does not just happen. It is induced by various causes. After all, it is your body's way of reacting to things it finds harmful. Some common causes of inflammation include:

Stress

Stress puts your body on high alert. It enables you to fight-or-flight whenever you are in danger. However, when your body releases adrenaline, it puts stress in your organs. For example, your heart rate increases and you start sweating or even trembling. When stress is temporary, the stress hormone will definitely come in handy to relieve the situation.

But if you are constantly stressed out, the emotional and physical toil on your body becomes too much as your body strives to mitigate all the symptoms of stress. An increased level of the stress hormone 'cortisol' is the one responsible for bringing about an inflammatory response. When you are stressed, you will exhibit symptoms like:

- Headaches
- Aches and pains
- Tense muscles
- Low energy
- Rapid heartbeat

Anti-Inflammatory Diet

- Chest pain
- Frequent cold and infection
- Insomnia
- Nervousness
- Cold or sweaty hands
- Dry mouth
- Difficulty swallowing
- Grinding teeth
- Clenched jaw
- Upset stomach – nausea, constipation, diarrhea
- Acne
- Eczema
- Hair loss
- Obesity
- Cardiovascular disease

All these symptoms put a considerable strain on your body and compromise your immune system. Furthermore, if stress is left unchecked, it will lead to other negative effects.

Psychological stress affects your body's ability to effectively regulate the inflammatory response. It is associated with diseases such as heart disease, depression and various infectious diseases. It weakens your immune system. If you are stressed, you will become susceptible to things such as the common cold. Thus, you should find healthy ways to de-stress. This will lessen inflammation.

Pathogens

Pathogens are another cause of inflammation. Pathogens are basically any agent that causes disease and they exist all around us. Pathogens such as fungus, parasites, bacteria, viruses and mold <u>trigger inflammation</u> when they invade the human body.

Your body induces a natural immune response by attracting white blood cells to the area. These cells work to engulf the pathogens and render them inactive. However, if pathogens such as bacteria and viruses multiply faster than your body can deal with them, then the infection turns into <u>disease</u> and this enhances the inflammatory response as your body struggles to repair the damage. As such, it would be wise to take care of your body, observe hygiene and keep up with your health checks.

Toxins

Toxins cause havoc in the body. They are poisonous. They work to disrupt hormones, damage organs and tissues, create autoimmunity, cause inflammation and suppress the immune system. <u>Chemical toxicity</u> has been linked to various inflammatory states such as lupus, hepatitis, scleroderma and nephritis.

In order to heal your body, you need to minimize your exposure to toxins. Toxins can be found in the air you breathe, the water you drink and the food you eat. They can also be found in medication, cleaning products, beauty products, mercury fillings, PVC containers and cigarette smoke.

It is important to note that toxins build up in your body over time. Thus, the more toxic products you are exposed to, the greater the buildup. Things such as air pollutants, pesticides, household chemicals, herbicides, food additives and perfumes can all increase the likelihood of inflammation.

Remember, inflammation is basically your body's response to anything it deems harmful. Toxins do not belong in your body and hence, your body reacts to them by inducing inflammation. Stay away from such things.

But there's another cause of inflammation that we want to focus on. This is your diet.

Chapter 3: Diet And Inflammation

We cannot talk about causes of inflammation without talking about diet. Diet causes a two-fold problem as far as chronic inflammation is concerned. First, if you follow an unhealthy diet, your body will not have the nutrients and antioxidants it needs to fight inflammation and heal itself. Secondly, if you follow an unhealthy diet, your body will be overburdened as it tries to get rid of the useless and harmful substances you're feeding it.

Lifestyle diseases such as diabetes are fueled by low-grade inflammation, which is in turn fueled by low dietary fiber, poor nutrition and living a sedentary life. It is no wonder that physicians call for dietary changes once an individual is affected by pre-diabetes or diabetes.

Another food product you should be on the lookout for is Trans fatty acid. This type of fat has been linked to systematic inflammation and predicts the risks of getting diseases such as diabetes and coronary artery disease. Other health issues such as obesity are also linked to inflammation components. This component is impacted by diet-induced increases in 'arachidonic acid'.

Additionally, certain foods cause your body to react by secretion of chemicals that induce an inflammatory response. For example, sugar is known to trigger cytokines. These are pro-inflammatory molecules that work to fan the flames of inflammation. As such, you would want to stay away from foods with high sugar content if you want to guard against inflammation.

Overall, as far as inflammation is concerned, the foods you eat can reduce or enhance inflammation. Some foods are anti-inflammatory and some foods are pro-inflammatory. Pro-inflammatory foods include foods such as:

- Sugary drinks
- White bread
- Processed meats
- White pasta
- Gluten
- Trans fat
- Vegetable oil
- Soybean oil
- Processed snacks such as crackers and chips
- Candy, Cookies and Cakes
- Excess alcohol

You should make it a point to minimize intake of foods that enhance inflammation.

Remember, your body can only heal itself if it has the right tools to do so. If you get rid of causes of inflammation, you are minimizing your body's enemies and lessening the chances of inflammation to occur in the first place.

Moreover, if you eat foods that are good for you, you're giving your body all the ammunition it needs to fight inflammation. This is why the anti-inflammatory diet exists. If you follow it, you will boost your immune system, keep disease at bay and enhance your energy levels and this will enrich your life.

Before we look at *how the foods that make up the anti-inflammatory diet work to fight inflammation*, let's first see *the specific health benefits of addressing the inflammation* in the first place i.e. how this diet can generally improve your life, with special focus on boosting energy, and improving the overall mental and physical health.

The Benefits Of The Anti-Inflammatory Diet

Maintains the brain's health and longevity

The natural process of aging involves a normal brain degeneration process and progressive cognitive decline -and we all know that. What few of us know is that we have the ability to reduce the rate at which our brains degenerate or get impaired by addressing one of their main contributors, which is the inflammatory chemicals.

Inflammatory chemicals in the body increase with age, causing brain inflammation- as this report published in the Journal of Therapeutic Advances in Chronic Disease asserts; not only does brain inflammation contribute to progressive brain damage, it also affects the day to day performance of the brain negatively.

https://www.drperlmutter.com/study/cognitive-dysfunction-aging-role-inflammation/

One of the most important mechanisms that correlates brain inflammation and brain damage or decline and performance is blood sugar. I mentioned earlier that glucose triggers the release of certain cytokines that increase inflammation in the body. As it turns out, that is not the only thing that happens when your glucose levels are high.

According to research, even a mild elevation in blood sugar increases the blood sugar's ability to attach to proteins in a process known as glycation. As more proteins become glycated, inflammatory chemicals in the body increase, resulting to brain decline. The brain tissue basically gets destroyed slowly, putting you at risk of further problems like Parkinson's and Alzheimer's disease.

As the inflammation gets worse, you also experience brain fog, depression, increased mental depression, anxiety and indecisiveness, which has little to do with the normal aging process. This is why the anti-inflammatory diet is designed to ensure your sugar intake is low and you are getting your energy from complex and high-fiber carbohydrates to minimize the levels of blood sugar in your blood stream at any given time.

The brain neurotransmitters

Most of us have accepted that memory problems and sometimes feelings of depression, agitation and insomnia are part of the normal aging process, but still don't understand why certain people still have better memory, low anxiety and depression, and sleep well in their old age.

If you've been one of the people wondering how that happens, you need to keep in mind that inflammation negatively affects various brain neurotransmitters as well. For instance, it decreases serotonin, which causes memory problems, anxiety and depression. It also inhibits the secretion of a hormone known as melatonin, which helps us create what is known as the 'sleep-wake cycle' or the circadian rhythm, which generally leads to insomnia.

The levels of another hormone known as dopamine also reduces and that's when you start experiencing agitation and anxiety. Glutamate, an excitatory neurotransmitter also increases and in turn, anxiety levels increase. This might be a minor effect considering what excess glutamate can really do (for instance, it can kill your brain cells).

As anxiety increases, so does your susceptibility to depression, which in turn causes the impairment of a prominent cell in the brain known as astrocyte that gives leeway to the inflammation process.

As you can see, there's so much you get to gain by adopting an anti-inflammatory diet in terms of maintaining the health of your brain and averting problems that have long been thought to be caused by aging. When your brain becomes healthy and fine, you feel good, and your life becomes generally better. Just imagine a life without so much mental exhaustion, brain fog, memory problems, depression, anxiety, insomnia and so forth. I don't know what that means for you but if you ask me, that means a good, productive life!

Boosts your energy levels

Did you know that inflammation might be the biggest culprit in your tiredness, lack of energy, or general feelings of lethargy and sluggishness? Today, there are many studies that have been conducted that clearly link fatigue and inflammation.

For instance, the two studies below, both done by the National Institute of Health, show that people suffering from chronic fatigue usually have more inflammation blood markers, which includes one known as the C-reactive protein and pro-inflammatory cytokines.

https://www.ncbi.nlm.nih.gov/pubmed/18031285'

https://www.ncbi.nlm.nih.gov/pubmed/19111923

That means that if you are always tired, sluggish and poor in mental performance, you are most probably suffering from inflammation. Please read more on that from the resource below.

https://www.ncbi.nlm.nih.gov/pmc/articles/PMC2657165/

Also, as this interesting NIH research suggests, inflammation can really have its way with your nervous system and brain very easily and make you feel fatigued all the time.

https://www.ncbi.nlm.nih.gov/pubmed/21334376

Bear in mind that when you suffer from chronic fatigue, the activation of the basal ganglia (this is the reward center of your brain) is significantly reduced (this is supported by a study that was published in PlOS ONE back in May 2014).

https://journals.plos.org/plosone/article?id=10.1371/journal.pone.0098156

In the aforementioned study, inflammation was concluded to be the main cause of the reduced activation after studying a group of individuals with chronic fatigue syndrome.

You might never get to the level of suffering from chronic fatigue but you can address your problem early before you make another step towards that direction. The anti-inflammatory diet is one of the surest ways to reduce the inflammation right from the nervous system and brain to ensure you stay energetic and active.

It assists you lose weight and manage or prevent type 2 diabetes

I'm sure you've heard of the *"diabesity" (*diabetes + obesity) epidemic which is said to be one of the biggest modern world problems. Unsurprisingly, inflammation has been a key contributing factor to this problem.

When the fat cells in the body get inflamed, something known as insulin resistance is created (insulin resistance is a condition where your body is not able to respond to insulin well and thus, it's job of carrying glucose out of the bloodstream to the cells for energy is not done effectively). This can lead to, among other problems, diabetes type 2 and weight gain and this is well researched and documented in the resources below:

http://www.jbc.org/content/277/52/50230.full

http://diabetes.diabetesjournals.org/content/52/8/2097.full?ijkey=c30ecf67b38ac20bc59ecf06ac0a8cbb539532fc

The thing is, when insulin in your body is not able to function properly, your cells become starved of the glucose and as a result, you eat more and more (since a part of you sort of perceives the situation as a lack of enough glucose/food in your body) and predictably, most of what you crave in such instances is sugary food.

Secondly, when your brain is inflamed, there is a high chance that it will begin resisting a chemical known as leptin, which, through a brain part known as hypothalamus, balances your appetite and metabolism. This resistance to leptin affects your metabolism negatively and you start gaining weight.

You also have to consider the fact that as you add weight, some fat cells in your body sometimes expand beyond their capacity in efforts to store the additional calories as fat. Almost simultaneously, they turn on inflammation, adding to the one that is already present, which not only makes these cells warehouses of fat storage but factories of inflammation as well. This is the reason why the most ideal diet here is one that can help you lose weight and fight inflammation at the same time.

By losing weight, your fat cells will return to their normal sizes and turn off signals that contribute to chronic inflammation.

Just to give you some evidence, let me mention that some time ago, the study below was done on this topic and it gave a clear link between chronic inflammation and weight gain.

https://www.ncbi.nlm.nih.gov/pmc/articles/PMC5079008/

The study's participants were monitored for a period of about nine years and factors like weight gain and the levels of a component known as C-reactive protein (that appears when the immune system is activated) in the blood. The researchers conclusively found that weight increase was heavily and linearly associated with increase in inflammation. By linear, I mean that the more an individual added weight, the more the levels of C-reactive protein in the blood increased.

Type 2 diabetes

When you stop responding to insulin properly as a consequence of systemic inflammation, you'd expect that the pancreas (the organ that produces insulin) will struggle to produce more and more insulin to try and keep the blood sugar levels under control and feed the body cells. That's exactly what happens. Over time, the pancreas becomes unable to produce the required amount of insulin (even though your blood is flooded with the hormone) as the pancreatic beta cells begin wearing out (as the insulin resistance worsens).

In the long run, the insulin your body is producing becomes too little to do anything, your system becomes flooded with glucose and you suffer from pre-diabetes and then type 2 diabetes eventually.

Let's now look at the foods you can eat on the anti-inflammatory diet.

Chapter 4: Vegetables For Fighting Inflammation

Vegetables should make up the core of the anti-inflammatory diet. They are rich in carotenoids and flavonoids and as such, they have the anti-inflammatory and antioxidants properties needed to fight inflammation and heal your body.

You should eat a minimum of 4-5 servings of vegetables each day. A serving is equal to a half-cup of cooked vegetables or about 2 cups of uncooked salad greens. When selecting your vegetables, try to go for a mixture of vegetables. Some vegetables you should eat include:

Green Leafy Vegetables

Green leafy vegetables enhance T-Bet in the immune system. This is a gene that plays a role in immune-related functions as far as the bowel is concerned. The gene also initiates ILCs- innate lymphoid cells. These cells prevent cancerous growth, maintain a balance between inflammation and cell immunity, protect your body against pathogenic infections and enhance the tolerance to substances that are inflammatory.

Green leafy vegetables have some of the highest levels of nutrients and antioxidants. They are basically designed to fight disease and inflammation. You can eat dark leafy greens such as kale, spinach, Swiss chard and collard greens or, cruciferous vegetables such as cauliflower, broccoli, bok choy, cabbage, kale and Brussels sprouts. You can also eat onions, peas and salad greens.

Broccoli

Broccoli is one vegetable that deserves its own mention when it comes to the fight against inflammation. It is rich in phytonutrients. One such phytonutrient happens to be sulforaphane. This phytonutrient has awesome anti-inflammatory properties and is at the forefront of fighting carcinogens.

Tomato

Tomatoes are nightshade vegetables that are high in phytonutrients. They contain phytonutrients such as flavonoids, carotenoids and anthocyanin. They also contain carotene and lycopene. These carotenoids act as antioxidants. Lycopene, in particular, is a powerful antioxidant. Its work is to scavenge free radicals and eradicate oxidative stress. This translates to reduced inflammation. Another thing that lycopene does is delays aging as well as improves cellular integrity. It also reduces the risk of cancers.

But what about anthocyanins?

Well, anthocyanins are the ones responsible for giving tomatoes their color. This phytochemical has excellent antioxidant and anti-inflammatory properties and works well to combat cancer and improve heart health. You can eat tomatoes in salads and sandwiches or you can add them to your food as you cook. You can also blend them and take them as a drink. This will ensure you get your share of these excellent phytonutrients.

Pepper

Pepper or chili is known for its heat. It gives food that extra kick and intensity. But there is another good reason you should eat pepper. This is because it contains capsaicin. This chemical gives it its pungency and provides it with its health benefits.

Capsaicin does a good job of inhibiting NF-kB. This is an inflammatory chemical. Buy not only does pepper inhibit this chemical but it also produces an anti-inflammatory effect.

Another way pepper produces an anti-inflammatory effect is by acting as a regional anesthesia. It degenerates nociceptor nerve endings and thus brings relief to inflamed areas.

It is no wonder that capsaicin is one of the ingredients in various creams, ointments and oils that are used topically to relieve pain and inflammation. You can use such products to find relief from muscle sores, arthritis and neuropathic pain.

Beets

Beetroot is another vegetable that can be used to fight inflammation. It is packed with nutrients and antioxidants that treat inflammation. It also has betaines. This bioactive compound is termed as cardio-protective. It works to block homocysteine in the blood. This chemical is linked to cardiac diseases. It harms the blood vessels whereas beetroot juice has been shown to actually reduce blood pressure.

Despite its benefits, many people do not like how beetroot tastes. However, this should not discourage you from eating beetroot. You can make it into a juice to make it more palatable or, you can hide it in other foods to mask the taste. The important thing is to include it in your anti-inflammatory diet.

Overall, you need to increase your intake of vegetables. Vegetables will provide you with all the nutrients and antioxidants you need to fight inflammation and repair your body. You can eat fresh or frozen vegetables.

Chapter 5: Fruits That Fight Inflammation

Fruits are well-known for their nutritional value. They contain various nutrients and antioxidants that are useful in fighting disease. As such, you need to eat 3-4 servings of fruits daily. A serving is basically one medium fruit. Some fruits you can eat include:

Avocado

Avocado gets its anti-inflammatory properties from persenone A. This component works to fight chemicals such as cyclooxygenase and oxide synthase. In particular, avocado is good when it comes to combating inflammation linked to cancer. As such, you should add it to your regular diet. Avocados are generally easy to find especially when they are in season. However, they can take awhile to ripen. Also, if you're not careful, they may end up going bad rather quickly once they ripen.

You can eat an avocado by itself or make guacamole by adding onions and tomatoes. You can also add some slices to your salad if you wish. Keep in mind that it oxidizes rather quickly once you remove the pit. Thus, you should only prepare it when you are ready to eat it.

Pineapple

Pineapples contain bromelain. This enzyme gives it its properties. One of the properties happens to be anti-inflammatory. It is said that bromelain action is similar to

NSAID acetaminophen and similar drugs when it comes to combating inflammation and pain in arthritis.

Arthritis can be quite painful and anything that can help relieve that pain is welcome. As such, you need to make sure you buy a ripe pineapple but not one that is overly ripe. You can blend the pineapple and drink it as a juice if you wish.

Berries and Cherries

Berries and cherries are high in antioxidants and Vitamin C. They have phytonutrients called anthocyanins. These phytonutrients are especially high in fruits such as cherries, raspberries and strawberries. Such fruits contain anthocyanins 1 and 2.

These phytonutrients are anti-inflammatory in nature and they work well to guard the heart and reduce the risk of diseases such as cancer. The good thing about berries is that they are often affordable and easy to find. You can eat them as they are or add them to your salads or even smoothies. When selecting berries, you should go for fresh ones that have no blemishes. Such berries will serve you well.

One thing to note about fruits is that some of them tend to be high in sugars. Thus, you should not overindulge in such fruits. As much as possible, you should eat your fruits instead of drinking them. If you want to make a fruit juice, you need to ensure that you keep the fiber as it will keep you fuller and it will be better for your gut health.

Chapter 6: Drinks

It's important to keep yourself well-hydrated as you embrace the anti-inflammatory diet. You can drink:

Tea

Tea is often used to treat patients suffering from arthritis as it helps preserve bone and cartilage. Black, green and white teas are rich in polyphenols. These are compounds with strong anti-inflammatory effects. Green and white teas have the highest amount if such compounds. Green tea, in particular, contains epigallocatechin3-gallate (EGCG). This active ingredient is said to be 100 times stronger than both Vitamin C and Vitamin E in terms of antioxidant activity. Thus, you will benefit greatly from drinking green tea. Black tea contains theaflavins. These antioxidants fight inflammation. Thus, although black tea is not as great as green tea, it too can help you reduce inflammation.

Bone broth

Bone broth should not be neglected in the fight against inflammation. Once you simmer the bones, you extract and break down their nutrients and collagen. One of the broken down material happens to be glucosamime. This is something that is often sold as a supplement for joint pain and arthritis.

But it is not the only useful substance in the fight against inflammation. You can also gain a lot from the stock. It is rich in anti-inflammatory amino acids such as proline and glycine. It also has gelatin and as such, it can help you repair your gut lining. This in turn will work to help you with the anti-inflammatory microbes. It does take some time to prepare bone broth but the benefits are definitely worth it.

Water

Water cannot be compared to any other drink. It's in a class of its own because without it, life ceases to exist. One thing it does so well is flush out toxins. This is very useful in the fight against inflammation.

As you've already seen, toxins lead to inflammation. Thus, getting rid of them is a good thing.

Another way that water helps in the fight against inflammation is by keeping the joints well lubricated. This prevents undue strain and can help prevent gout attacks. You should embrace the practice of drinking water throughout the day.

Red Wine

Red wine is another drink that is usually touted for its health benefits. It contains resveratol. This compound gives it its anti-inflammatory properties. It is linked to the reduced risk of knee injury.

In terms of consumption, women should drink one glass of red wine daily whereas men can drink up to two glasses daily. However, you need to be cautious when drinking wine. If you drink more than you should, you will negate the anti-inflammatory benefits. Also, you don't need to drink wine if you're not used to it or if you have a problem with alcohol. You can stick to the other anti-inflammatory drinks for your own peace of mind.

Your drink of choice should be water but other drinks can supplement it. However, don't make the practice of adding sugar or other harmful artificial sweeteners to your drinks. Remember, you are trying to fight inflammation not introduce pro-inflammatory products to your body.

Chapter 7: Great Protein And Fats For Dealing With Inflammation

Proteins

Protein is an important part of your diet. But you need to eat healthy protein that will ease inflammation. Some great sources of protein for dealing with inflammation include:

Hemp seeds

Hemp seeds are good for you. This is because they contain all 20 amino acids. Since they have a high ration of these essential fatty acids, they serve as a great anti-inflammatory food. As such, you can use hemp seeds to reduce pain and inflammation. They are especially used in reducing skeletal and muscle inflammation. You can add such seeds to your soups and salads if you wish. The idea is to make them a regular part of your diet.

Walnuts

Walnuts are known for their omega-3 fatty acids. However, they also contain polyphenols and antioxidant phytonutrients. This combination of omega-3s, phytonutrients and polyphenols works well in combating inflammation. However, you need to be careful when eating walnuts as some people are allergic to them. You should monitor how you feel once you eat it to ensure that it is actually helping you to reduce inflammation rather than adding on to your health issues.

Fatty Fish

Oily fish are loaded with omega-3 fatty acids and omega-6s. These fatty acids work to increase eicosapentaenoic acid, an acid that fights inflammation. Fatty fish such as salmon, trout and tuna can help reduce inflammation brought about by diseases such as IBD, arthritis and cardiovascular disease. Thus, it would be good to eat fatty fish at least 1-2 times each week.

Steam the fish for best results but to not deep fry them as this will greatly lessen its benefits. Also, you need to get your fish from a reputable vendor and ensure it is not contaminated with mercury to avoid other health issues.

Please note that fish is not the only source of protein you can enjoy. You can also eat 1-2 servings of beans and other legumes each week. This will make the diet more interesting for you. But as you have your choice of protein, you should remember not to go overboard in your consumption of protein. Moderation is the key.

Healthy Fats

In addition to protein, healthy fats are important too. Healthy fats can help you fight inflammation and they are also useful in distributing fat-soluble nutrients. Healthy fats sources include:

Olive oil

Olive oil is often touted for its health benefits but there is one thing that makes it stand out from other oils. This is a compound known as oleocanthal. This compound is unique to extra virgin olive oils. Such oils have more phenolic compounds and are unrefined. Thus, they have the ability to significantly affect inflammation.

You can use olive oil to reduce cartilage damage and joint damage. Its anti-inflammatory compound works similarly to ibuprofen. It effectively prevents the production of COX-1 and COX-2 enzymes. These are pro-inflammatory enzymes that harm the body.

You should make it a point to use olive oil whenever you cook your food. You can also add it to your salads and soups. Remember, fat is part of the macro nutrients your body uses for energy. There is no harm in increasing the amount of healthy fats you eat each day. You should aim to eat at least 30% of fats each day when you are on the anti-inflammatory diet.

Coconut Oil

Coconut oil is also known for its various health benefits. Many people use it to cook their food or they apply it on their hair and skin. But you can specifically use it for its anti-inflammatory properties.

Actually, coconut oil is often used to treat acute inflammation. It is topically applied to injured areas or areas with infections. You can use coconut oil to ease the pain and inflammation caused by things such as sunburn or insect bites.

You can use it the way it is or in salves and creams. Coconut oil tends to have a strong taste. As such, you may want to mask that taste by adding it to your food or drink. However, if you have no issue with the taste, you can make it a point to drink it directly.

Obviously, you will get your share of fats from other foods you eat. However, you should take at least 5-7 teaspoons of oil each day. Every time you eat a salad, drizzle it with some oil instead of going for unhealthy dressings. Try as much as possible to eat healthy fats.

Chapter 8: Whole Grains That Can Address Inflammation

For a while, carbohydrates have been touted as the energy. However, the bad carbohydrates are the processed ones while whole grains are actually quite good for you.

Whole grains include foods such as wild rice, brown rice, barley, quinoa and buckwheat grouts. Such grains take longer to digest. As such, they reduce spikes in blood sugar. Such spikes often promote inflammation. Thus, it would be best to stick to whole grains.

You also need to stay away from gluten. Things like whole-wheat bread and other wheat flour products can worsen inflammation. A great whole grain that you should try is oats.

Raw oats are well-known resistant starch. Thus means that they remain undigested as they pass through your gut. However, while they don't feed you, they do feed the healthy gut bacteria. This is important as it leads to such bacteria producing a fatty acid. This in turn leads to efficient fat oxidation called butyrate. High levels of butyrate in your body lead to a reduction in inflammation. It also works to reduce insulin resistance. Thus, you'll end up losing weight and reducing issues such as bloating. You can make overnight oats and add berries, nuts, dark chocolate and a bit of cinnamon. All these foods reduce inflammation and are good for you.

Remember, highly processed foods not only cause inflammation but they also lead to issues such as obesity that are attributed to inflammation. Eat whole grains for your own good.

Chapter 9: Herbs And Spices

Herbs and spices should feature prominently in your day-to-day diet. Some herbs and spices you can use include:

Ginger

Ginger tea is a favorite drink for many people and for good reason. It contains compounds known as gingerols. These compounds are antibacterial, anti-inflammatory, antioxidant and anti-disease. They are the ones responsible for giving ginger its health benefits.

According to studies, gingerols work to block several enzymes and genes that promote inflammation. This action not only reduces inflammation but also inhibits joint swelling. In order to get the most out of these compounds, you should stick to fresh ginger. You can grate up the ginger root and place it in a mesh bag and then steep in hot water to make ginger tea.

Garlic

Garlic has been used for years to fight the common cold. This is because it contains allicin. This compound works to block enzymes that enhance viral and bacterial infections.

However, cold-fighting is not the only use for garlic. You can also use it to fight inflammation. This is especially true of aged garlic extracts. Such extracts are known to suppress inflammatory markers where chronic inflammation is concerned.

Aged-garlic supplements contain a high concentration of the bioavailable compounds and are thus better for fighting inflammation. Still, you can also use fresh garlic to reduce inflammation. But before you do, you need to make sure you crush it well as this will stimulate allicin production.

Cinnamon

Cinnamon is a well-known warming spice. It comes in handy during cold days. But there is another good reason you should add it to your regular diet. It is good for fighting inflammation.

Cinnamon contains bio-active compounds such as cinnamylacetate, cinnamyl alcohol and also cinnamaldehyde. These compounds give it its health benefits. Cinnamaldehyde, in particular, works to attack inflammatory pathways. It is anti-inflammatory in nature. Its act of inhibiting inflammatory pathways makes it useful in preventing diseases such as Alzheimer's disease, Parkinson's disease, meningitis and multiple sclerosis. In general, cinnamon inhibits inflammation in the brain and this contributes to brain health.

Turmeric

Indian saffron, commonly known as turmeric, ranks amongst the best anti-inflammatory foods. This is because it has an active compound known as curcumin. This compound gives it its color and makes for a potent anti-inflammatory agent.

Curcumin also has antioxidant properties. According to studies, curcumin works to shut down COX-1 and 5-LOX. These are pro-inflammatory enzymes. Thus, by inhibiting the activation of such enzymes, curcumin is useful in preventing heart disease, liver damage and cognitive inflammation. It is also useful in reducing pain and joint inflammation. People suffering from arthritis would do well to add turmeric to their diet.

Herbs and spices really provide you with a variety of tastes but they may take time to get used to. Start small and gradually increase your intake of these anti-inflammatory foods. Make it a point to have them in your vicinity whenever you cook or sit down to eat. This way, it will be easier to reach for them and add them to your food. If they are hidden in drawers, you may end up remembering them only after you are done eating and this will not aide your fight against inflammation.

Now that you have a better idea of what the anti-inflammatory diet looks like, let's see how you can bring together all those foods to make delicious meals.

The Anti-Inflammatory Diet Recipes
Breakfast Recipes
Amaranth Porridge with Roasted Pears

Serves 2

Ingredients

Porridge

¼ teaspoon salt

1 cup 2% milk

1/2 cup water

½ cup uncooked amaranth

Pears

1 teaspoon maple syrup

1/2 teaspoon ground cinnamon

1/8 teaspoon ground nutmeg

1 large pear

1/4 teaspoon ground ginger

1/8 teaspoon ground clove

Topping

2 tablespoons pecan pieces

Anti-Inflammatory Diet

1 cup plain 0% Greek yogurt, for serving

1 teaspoon pure maple syrup

Directions

Preheat your oven to 400 degrees. Meanwhile, drain the amaranth and rinse it.

Mix it with the water, milk and salt and bring it to a boil before reducing it to a simmer.

Cover it and give it 25 minutes to simmer until the amaranth softens but some liquid remains.

Remove it from the heat and let it sit for between 5 – 10 minutes so that the amaranth thickens.

Add some more milk for the texture to thin out if you want.

Toss a teaspoon of maple syrup with the pieces of pecan and roast until they are properly toasted and the syrup has fully dried, for between 10 and 15 minutes. The pecans will be fragrant when they are done and crisp, as they cool.

Now dice the pears and then toss with the spices and one teaspoon of maple syrup.

Add these ingredients to a roasting pan and roast for about 15 minutes, until the pears become tender.

Add ¾ of the roasted pears in the porridge and stir. Now add the yoghurt to two bowls and then the porridge nicely over it, and top with the rest of the pear pieces and roasted pecans.

Whole 30 Sweet Potato Protein Breakfast Bowl

Serves 1

Ingredients

1 pre-baked small sweet potato

1 small banana, sliced

1/4 cup blueberries

Cacao nibs

Hemp hearts

1 serving protein powder

1/4 cup raspberries

Optional toppings

Chia seeds

Favorite nut/seed butter

Directions

Flesh out the sweet potato if it's not already prepared and mash it in a small bowl with a fork.

Stir in the protein powder until they combine well.

Add a layer of the banana slices, blueberries and raspberries.

Add your favorite toppings and enjoy. You can eat it cold or warm- your choice.

Turkey Apple Breakfast Hash (AIP)

Serves 5 portions (as a breakfast)

Ingredients

The meat

½ teaspoon dried thyme

1 lb. ground turkey

Sea salt, to taste

1 tablespoon coconut oil

½ teaspoon cinnamon

The hash

1 large or 2 small zucchini

2 cups of cubed frozen sweet potato or butternut squash

2 cups your preferred greens (e.g. spinach)

¾ teaspoon of ginger, powdered

½ teaspoon turmeric

1 tablespoon coconut oil

Sea salt, to taste

1 onion

½ cup shredded carrots

Anti-Inflammatory Diet

1 large apple, peeled, cored, and chopped

1 teaspoon cinnamon

½ teaspoon garlic powder

½ teaspoon dried thyme

Directions

Add one tablespoon of coconut oil to a skillet and heat it over medium –high heat.

Add the turkey and cook until it turns brown. Season it with thyme, cinnamon and a pinch of sea salt and move to the plate.

Add the rest of the coconut oil to the same skillet, add the onion and sauté for 2-3 minutes, or until softened.

Add the carrots, zucchini, frozen squash and apple and cook for 4-5 minutes, or until the veggies soften.

Add the spinach and stir until it wilts.

Add the cooked turkey, seasonings and salt and then turn off the heat.

Enjoy immediately (fresh and straight from the skillet) or allow it to cool in your refrigerator over a period of 6 days (the hash can keep up to the sixth day if you keep it in a sealed container and cool it).

Maple-Baked Rice Porridge Recipe With Fruit

Serves 2

Ingredients

½ cup brown rice

Pinch of cinnamon

Sliced fruit, like berries, plums, pears or cherries

½ teaspoon pure vanilla extract

2 tablespoons pure maple syrup

Pinch of salt (optional)

Directions

Preheat your oven to 400 degrees.

Add 1 cup of water and the rice to a pot and set it over medium-high heat.

When it boils, add the cinnamon and vanilla extract and stir.

Cover well and reduce the heat to medium low.

Let it simmer for 10 to 15 minutes (you can also follow the package directions if you are using a rice variety that takes more time to cook).

Stir the rice and divide it between two heat-safe bowls.

Add a tablespoon of maple syrup to each bowl and any sliced fruit you like. If desired, sprinkle some salt.

Bake the dish for 10 to 15 minutes or until the maple syrup bubbles and the fruit starts caramelizing.

Serve immediately and enjoy!

Lunch Recipes

Deep Dish Falafel Pizza

Ingredients

Falafel Crust

3/4 cup of cooked chickpeas

1 cup fresh coriander

3 tablespoons tahini

2 tablespoons cumin

2 cloves of garlic

1/3 cup of oats, millet or flour

1 small red onion

1 cup fresh mint

3 tablespoons ground chia or flax

2 tablespoons coriander powder

Beet hummus

1/2 cup cooked chickpeas

2 tablespoons tahini

Basil, oregano, and other herbs, as desired

1 small beet, boiled

1 cloves garlic

Sliced vegetables, as desired

Tahini cheese sauce:

Nutritional yeast, to taste

2 tablespoons tahini

Directions

Preheat your oven to 390 degrees F. and line your deep pie dish or cake pan with baking paper.

Make the base

Pulse all the crust ingredients in a food processor until they're all well integrated. Spread the mixture on the lower sides and bottom of your pie dish/cake pan and bake for 20 minutes in your oven.

Make the beet humus

Pulse all the ingredients in your food processor until they form a smooth mixture.

Remove the beet hummus and add all the sliced veggies to the hummus. Mix properly.

When the falafel crust feels dry to the touch, take it out of the oven.

Pour the beet hummus over the crust evenly and take it back to the oven. Bake for about 40 minutes.

Make the cheese sauce

Combine all the ingredients and drizzle over the pizza when the baking completes. Slice and serve.

Enjoy!

Sweet Potato 'Rice' Casserole

Serves 3

Ingredients

The pesto

2 1/2 cups basil leaves, packed

1/4 cup olive oil (or less if you like it thicker)

5 cranks of a peppercorn grinder

3 tablespoons pine nuts

5 cranks of a sea salt grinder

1 large garlic clove, minced

The rest

2 cups small broccoli florets

Pepper, to taste

1 1/2 cups shredded vegan mozzarella (optional)

1 large sweet potato, peeled

1/3 cup low-sodium vegetable broth

Directions

Preheat your oven to 400 degrees F.

Add all the pesto ingredients to a blender or food processor and process until smooth.

Then taste and adjust whatever needs to be adjusted.

Pout half the mixture out into a bowl and then add the broccoli.

Toss it until the broccoli is evenly coated with the pesto mixture.

Set the broccoli and the rest of the pesto aside.

Now spread out a thin layer of the pesto on the casserole and them a layer of the sweet potato rice.

Next, add the broccoli and them the rest of the rice over the broccoli to cover it.

Drizzle the rest of the pesto over the rice and then pour over the vegetable broth.

Add some pepper.

If you're using mozzarella, spread it over the rice evenly to cover it.

Use a tinfoil to cover the casserole.

Bake it for 40 minutes.

Serve when ready and enjoy.

Anti-Inflammatory Orange Chicken And Spinach Salad

Serves 4

Ingredients

4 large navel oranges

1/4 cup olive oil

1 tablespoon raw honey

2 tablespoons rice wine vinegar or cider vinegar

1/2 teaspoon salt and pepper

4 6oz. each of chicken breasts, boneless and skinless with the tenderloins removed

1 halved and sliced small red onion

1 bag (5-6oz.) baby spinach

Toasted sliced almonds to garnish, optional

Directions

Squeeze the juice from one orange (this makes ½ cup) and add it to a small bowl along with the vinegar, honey, pepper, three tablespoons of oil and salt.

Whisk the ingredients to combine.

Add five tablespoons of the juice mixture into a large zip lock bag.

Add the chicken and seal the bag.

Marinate at room temperature for 15 minutes.

Meanwhile, unpeel the other three oranges and remove their white pith.

Cut them into segments and put them in a medium-sized bowl.

Place a stovetop grill over medium high heat.

Remove the chicken from the marinade and grill it for 4-5 minutes on each side until it cooks through.

Transfer to a plate and cover it to retain its warmth.

Add the rest of the oil in a medium-sized skillet and set it over medium-high heat.

Add the onion and sauté for one minute. Add the rest of the juice mixture and cook for one more minute.

Remove the skillet from the heat and add the orange segments.

Put the spinach in a large bowl and toss it with half of the orange mixture.

Divide the spinach evenly among serving plates.

Put a chicken breast atop each one.

Spoon the rest of the orange mixture on top and sprinkle with almonds.

Enjoy!

Curried Red Lentil And Swiss Chard Soup

Serves 6

Ingredients

2 tablespoons olive oil

5 teaspoons curry powder

2 cups (about 14 oz.) dried red lentils

1 teaspoon salt

1 red or green jalapeño chili, stemmed and thinly sliced

1 large onion, thinly sliced

5 cups of vegetable broth

1/4 teaspoon ground red pepper (cayenne)

1 bunch Swiss chard, tough stalks removed, coarsely chopped

1 can (15-ounce) of rinsed and drained chickpeas

6 tablespoons of thick Greek yogurt, use 2 tablespoons of water to thin it a little

1 lime, cut into 6 wedges

Directions

Add the oil to a heavy sauce pan set over medium heat.

When it heats up, add the onion and cook, stirring often until it turns light golden, for about ten minutes.

Add red pepper and curry as you stir.

Add four cups of the chard and broth, increase the heat and while stirring, bring to a boil, until the chard wilts.

Add the chickpeas and lentils while stirring.

Reduce the heat to low and simmer, covered, for 16 – 18 minutes.

Only stir twice until the lentils become tender.

Now remove from the heat and puree about four cups of the soup (half the soup) in a food processor or blender.

Take back the puree to the pot.

Add the rest of the broth and salt while stirring and warm for 2 minutes over low heat.

Now divide the soup among six bowls and drizzle one tablespoon of the thinned yoghurt over each one of them.

Garnish with a few jalapeno slices and a wedge of lime.

Anti-Inflammatory Salad

Serves 4-6

Ingredients

24-28 oz. bag of sweet kale salad mix and nut/seed and dried fruit packet (e.g. Trader Joe's sweet kale salad mix)

1/3 can of extra virgin olive oil

1 tablespoon lemon juice

1 clove of garlic, grated

½ teaspoon sea salt

½ teaspoon sea salt

1 ½ can fresh blueberries

Turmeric Dressing

16oz. cooked, cooled, and peeled beets quartered or chopped

2 tablespoons apple cider vinegar

1 teaspoon turmeric

1 teaspoon fresh grated ginger

¼ teaspoon freshly ground black pepper

Directions

Combine all the ingredients together. If you want a smooth dressing, simply blend them together.

Anti-Inflammatory Diet

Divide the salad between the bowls and top with blueberries, beets, and seed/nut mixture.

Serve as is or drizzle with a dressing of your choice first.

Enjoy.

White Turkey Chili And Avocado

Serves 8

Ingredients

2 tablespoons extra-virgin olive oil

4 garlic cloves, minced

2 teaspoons ground cumin

1 teaspoon cayenne pepper

4 cups chicken broth

One 15-ounce can white beans

1 large white onion, diced

1 pound ground turkey

1 teaspoon ground coriander

Salt and freshly ground black pepper

One 15-ounce can corn kernels

1 avocado, diced

Directions

Add the olive oil to a large pot and set it over medium heat.

Sauté the onion until it turns translucent, which should take between 6 and 8 minutes.

Next, add the garlic and keep on cooking for one more minute, until fragrant.

Add the turkey and continue cooking until it fully cooks and is nicely browned, for between 5 and 7 minutes.

Next, add the coriander, cumin and cayenne then season with pepper and salt.

Cook for one or two minutes, until fragrant.

Add the broth while stirring, then reduce the heat to low, and let the soup simmer until it develops a good flavor, which should take 30 to 35 minutes.

Add the corn and beans while stirring, and simmer for 2 to 3 more minutes.

When ready, divide the chili into bowls and add 1 or 2 tablespoons of avocado on top.

Serve and enjoy!

Chicken and Snap Pea Stir-Fry

Serves 4

Ingredients

2 tablespoons vegetable oil

2 garlic cloves, minced

2½ cups snap peas

Salt and freshly ground black pepper

2 tablespoons rice vinegar

2 tablespoons sesame seeds, and a bit more for finishing

1 bunch scallions, thinly sliced

1 red bell pepper, thinly sliced

1¼ cups boneless skinless chicken breast, thinly sliced

3 tablespoons soy sauce

2 teaspoons Sriracha (optional)

3 tablespoons chopped fresh cilantro, plus more for finishing

Directions

Add the oil to a large sauté pan and heat it over medium heat.

Add the garlic and scallions and sauté them for a minute, until fragrant.

Add the snap peas and bell pepper and then sauté for 2-3 minutes, until they turn slightly tender.

Now add the chicken and cook it until it turns golden and fully cooked, for 4 to 5 minutes; the veggies should also be tender by then.

Now add the rice vinegar, soy sauce, sesame seeds and sriracha if you're using it and toss well to mix.

Let the mixture simmer for one to 2 minutes.

Now add the cilantro while stirring and then garnish with some extra sesame seeds and a sparkle of cilantro.

Serve and enjoy!

Smoked Salmon Salad With Green Goddess Dressing

Serves 4

Ingredients

1/2 cup of rinsed French green lentils

1/2 cup natural yoghurt

2 tablespoons chopped fresh chives

1 tablespoon salted baby capers, rinsed, drained

1/2 red onion, thinly sliced

Pinch of caster sugar

1/2 avocado, sliced

2 thinly sliced baby fennel bulbs with some fronds reserved

2 tablespoons of chopped fresh continental parsley, and some more leaves, to serve

1 tablespoon chopped fresh tarragon

1 teaspoon finely grated lemon rind

1 tablespoon fresh lemon juice

60g baby spinach

180g sliced salt-reduced smoked salmon

Directions

Add the lentils in boiling water and leave them to cook for 20 minutes, until tender and drain.

In the meantime, set a chargrill pan over high heat, and then spray the fennel slices with oil.

Cook them well on each side for 2 minutes or until tender.

Add the parsley, capers, chives, lemon rind, tarragon and yoghurt in a food processor and process until smooth, and then season the dish with pepper.

Add the juice, sugar, a pinch of salt and onion in a bowl and set aside for five minutes.

Drain.

Get a large bowl and add the lentils, spinach, fennel, avocado and onion.

Mix and divide it among the plates you're using.

Top the dish with salmon.

To serve, sprinkle with the remaining fennel fronds and some parsley, and drizzle with your favorite dressing (like the green goddess dressing).

Black Bean With Creamy Cashew Dressing

Serves 4

Ingredients

1 cup tri-colored quinoa, rinsed, drained

2 teaspoons ground cumin

1 red onion, finely chopped

2 teaspoons sweet paprika

2 zucchini, trimmed, cut into thin noodles

Thinly sliced long fresh red chili, to serve

2 1/3 cups water

2 teaspoons extra virgin olive oil

2 garlic cloves, crushed

400g can black beans, rinsed and drained

2 corncobs, cooked, kernels removed

Fresh coriander leaves, to serve

Coriander and cashew dressing

50g raw cashews, soaked in cold water for 3 hours

1 tablespoon extra-virgin olive oil

1/4 cup water

1 tablespoon lemon juice

2 tablespoons chopped fresh coriander

Ingredients

Add the two cups of water, 1 teaspoon of the cumin and quinoa in a saucepan and set it over medium heat.

Allow them to boil and then reduce the heat to low.

Cook for 12 minutes, covered, or until the water gets absorbed and the quinoa is nicely al dente.

Add the oil to a saucepan and heat it over medium heat.

Cook the onion for five minutes or until softened.

Now add the paprika, garlic and the rest of the cumin and cook while stirring for one minute, or until aromatic.

Add the rest of the water and then the black beans, and simmer for five minutes or until the water almost completely evaporates.

Mash the beans using a fork coarsely.

To dress, drain the cashews and add them to a food processor along with the lemon juice, coriander and oil until well integrated.

Add the water gradually until it becomes thick and creamy.

Now divide the bean mixture, quinoa, corn and zucchini among the bowls and drizzle with the dressing.

Finish by sprinkling some coriander and chili.

Serve and enjoy!

Anti-Inflammatory Diet

Puttanesca-Style Beans and Greens

Serves 6

Ingredients

3/4 cup pitted green olives

3 cups water

1/2 large yellow onion

6 tablespoons extra-virgin olive oil

4 anchovies, or 1-2 teaspoons anchovy paste (optional)

1 cup dried baby lima beans, soaked overnight

1 cup pitted kalamata olives

1/2 cup sun-dried tomatoes in olive oil (optional)

2 teaspoons capers

2 cups shredded greens (beet greens, dandelion greens, chard or kale all work well)

1 to 2 cloves garlic

One (6-inch) strip kombu (optional)

Directions

Add the water, kombu and lima beans to a large pot and bring to a boil over high heat.

Reduce the heat to medium low, then cover and simmer for about 40 minutes, or until the beans become tender.

Now drain the beans and throw away the kombu.

In the meantime, add the sun-dried tomatoes, olives, capers and onion to a blender or food processor and pulse until the mixture becomes coarsely chopped.

Now add two tablespoons of the oil to a skillet and set it over medium heat.

Sauté the olive mixture for five minutes, or until the onions just become translucent.

Now add the anchovies, garlic and the greens and sauté for 3-4 minutes.

Add the beans while stirring until well incorporated.

Serve the dish at room temperature or warm and enjoy.

Orecchiette Pasta with Kale Pesto

Serves 2

Ingredients

Ingredients

1 bunch fresh kale, roughly chopped

2 fresh sage leaves

1 cup toasted pine nuts

1 teaspoon Dijon mustard

½ lemon, juice only

2 cups orrechiette pasta

1 small bunch fresh basil

3 garlic cloves

2 tablespoon extra-virgin olive oil

½ teaspoon red chili flakes

Pinch of sea salt

Toasted pine nuts, fresh lemon juice and red chili flakes

Directions

Add the lemon juice, fresh greens, olive oil and garlic to a food processor and pulse a couple of times to get a nice mash.

Next, add the chili flakes, Dijon, pine nuts and salt and pulse a couple more times to combine.

Pour the mixture into a jar with a lid.

Add a layer of extra virgin olive oil over the pesto to help it store longer in the refrigerator.

Prepare the orrechiette according to the given instructions and transfer it to a large bowl; add three tablespoons of the pesto and mix properly to integrate.

Divide the dish into two bowls and garnish with red chili flakes and pine nuts and drizzle with olive oil and fresh lemon juice.

Serve warm and enjoy.

Loaded Sesame Ginger Salmon Salad

Serves 4

Ingredients

<u>The salmon</u>

1 lb. salmon, cut into four 4-ounce filets

Freshly cracked black pepper

Kosher salt

1 tablespoon olive oil

<u>The salad</u>

1 bunch fresh watercress

½ cup cilantro leaves

1 cup mango, small diced

1 avocado, sliced

½ cup chopped scallion leaves

1 cup cooked edamame

1 cup Persian cucumber, sliced

<u>Ginger vinaigrette</u>

2 clove garlic

1 tablespoons agave nectar

2 teaspoons soy sauce

3 tablespoon vegetable oil

2 inches of ginger, peeled and diced

¼ cup rice wine vinegar

1 teaspoons sesame oil

Kosher salt

Directions

Sprinkle the fish filets with pepper and salt

Add oil to a nonstick pan and set it over high heat.

When the oil heats up, add the salmon and cook it for 2-3 minutes.

Flip it and cook it for one more minute on the side with the skin.

Transfer the salmon to a plate.

Arrange the salad ingredients on a large plate then set aside.

Add the vinaigrette ingredients to a blender and puree until smooth.

Season with some kosher salt to taste.

Place the salmon on the salad and drizzle the dish using the ginger vinaigrette.

Desserts, Appetizers And Snacks

Low Carb Coconut Crunch

Serves 1 or 2

Ingredients

2 cups of unsweetened desiccated/ flaked coconut

1 teaspoon ground sea salt

4 tablespoons of coconut oil

1 tablespoons Chia seeds – optional

Directions

Pre-heat your oven to 180 degrees. Meanwhile, line your baking tray with aluminum foil.

Combine all the ingredients, making sure the coconut oil coats all the coconut flakes.

Bake the mixture in the oven for about five minutes, and take it out when it turns golden brown.

Make sure you check on it regularly because it does not take long to burn.

When you take it out of the oven, it will be resembling a course, unbound breadcrumb.

You can leave let it cool for one hour on the bench top and when it starts stiffening and binding together, pop it into the fridge to get a delicious coconut crunch ten minutes or so later.

Fried Plantains with Cinnamon

Serves 1

Ingredients

1 ripe plantain, peeled

1/4 teaspoon cinnamon

1 tablespoon ghee or coconut oil

Sea salt to taste

Directions

Slice the plantain into ¼ inch rounds and cut it diagonally.

Heat the coconut oil or ghee in a cast iron skillet set over medium-high heat and fry the plantains until they turn golden brown on each side.

That should take 2-3 minutes for each side.

Be careful because they can burn quite easily sprinkle some sea salt and cinnamon.

Two Ingredient Pumpkin Ice Cream

Serves 4

Ingredients

4 large ripe bananas (with black spots), frozen

Raw honey, non-irradiated cinnamon, pure maple syrup or chocolate chips

½ cup fresh or canned pumpkin puree

Directions

Add the pumpkin and frozen bananas to a blender and blend until creamy (if the bananas are not frozen, you will have to freeze the ice cream after you finish blending).

Taste; if desired, add maple syrup or any other sweetener.

You can also blend in chocolate chips and cinnamon if you want.

Serve immediately to obtain a soft texture or chill for four hours or more to get a firmer ice cream.

When you finally take the ice cream out of the freezer, give it about five minutes to sit at room temperature before digging in.

Homemade Pumpkin Applesauce

Serves 2

Ingredients

2lbs. apples, peeled, cored, and sliced

1 small lemon, juiced

1/3 cup pumpkin puree (if you want more pumpkin flavor, you can add 1/2 cup)

1 1/2 teaspoons ground cinnamon

1/2 cup water

Directions

Put all the apples into a sauce pan and add the lemon juice, water, cinnamon; stir.

Set the pan over medium heat and bring to a boil.

Reduce the heat and let the dish simmer for between 45 minutes and one hour; the apples should be very soft by then.

If you want your applesauce smoother, just pour the apples when they're ready into a blender and blend along with the pumpkin puree until smooth or until it reaches a desirable consistency.

If you want to have a chunkier sauce, simply stir in the pumpkin puree in with the apples.

Mash the apples using a potato masher until it attains a desirable consistency.

Refrigerate the leftovers in a container.

3-Ingredient Banana Pudding Recipe

Serves 1

Ingredients

1 ripe banana peeled

2 tablespoons chia seeds

1/4 cup full-fat coconut milk

Dash of vanilla extract (optional)

Directions

Add the coconut milk and banana to a food processor and process until smooth.

Next, add the chia seeds and process until well integrated.

Add the product into a container and freeze for one hour to allow the chia seeds to plump slightly.

You can also eat it right away if you want to have the seeds crunchy.

Anti-Inflammatory Diet

Slow Cooker Applesauce (without sugar)

Yields 1 1/2 quarts

Ingredients

10 medium to large apples, cored and roughly chopped (if desired, you can peel them as well)

1 cup water

2 cinnamon sticks

Ground cinnamon, for finishing

Directions

Add the chopped apples, cinnamon sticks and water to the bowl of a slow cooker and cook on low heat for 4-5 hours, covered, until the apples soften.

When the dish is ready, remove the cinnamon sticks and stir to break up the apples using a wooden spoon until it attains a desirable consistency to get a chunkier applesauce.

You can also transfer the apples to a food processor and pulse until smooth if you want a smooth applesauce.

Finish by adding ground cinnamon to taste.

Enjoy and store any leftovers in the fridge.

A warm applesauce is just as great as the cool applesauce though.

Turmeric Broccoli Chicken Roll Ups

Yields 8

Ingredients

Gourmet chicken roll ups.

One head of broccoli, sliced into eight long stalks

1 tablespoon minced fresh ginger

6 crimini mushrooms, sliced

1 teaspoon Himalayan or Celtic sea salt

1 heaping tablespoon coconut oil

4 boneless, skinless chicken breast halves

One 400 ml. tin full fat coconut milk

1 whole large clove garlic minced

1/2 large onion diced

1/2 teaspoon powdered turmeric

Directions

Preheat your oven to 350 degrees F and sauté the mushrooms and onions until the mushrooms turn golden brown and the onions translucent.

Reduce the heat to low and add some ginger and garlic then sauté without allowing the ginger to turn brown.

Now add the coconut milk, turmeric and salt and simmer to thicken a bit.

Steam the broccoli until it is almost fork tender.

In the meantime, put the chicken breast into a zip lock bag and pound it to a thickness of a quarter inch (you can also place it between two sheets of cling wrap).

<u>To assemble</u>

Place a spear of broccoli on the chicken to have the flower end lining up with one edge of the flattened chicken, and put a second spear to have the flower end lining up with the other edge (it's the same as putting shoes in a box end to end).

Now spoon one or two tablespoons of your prepared coconut milk sauce on top of the broccoli and tuck one chicken edge over the length of broccoli and roll it up.

If you want, pin it using toothpicks.

Slice through the middle so that in the end you have two equal halves of rolled up chicken- each with a flower of broccoli poking out of one end.

Out them in a baking dish, making sure to have the cut edge down and spoon the rest of the coconut milk sauce over the roll-ups.

Bake for half an hour at 350 degrees F.

When ready, serve and enjoy!

Anti-Inflammatory Diet

The Two-Week Meal Plan Table (Sample)

Week 1

	Sunday	Monday	Tuesday	Wednesday	Thursday	Friday	Saturday
Breakfast	Amaranth Porridge with Roasted Pears	Whole 30 Sweet Potato Protein Breakfast Bowl	Turkey Apple Breakfast Hash (AIP)	Maple-baked rice porridge recipe with fruit	Amaranth Porridge with Roasted Pears	Whole 30 Sweet Potato Protein Breakfast Bowl	Turkey Apple Breakfast Hash (AIP)
Lunch	Deep Dish Falafel Pizza	Anti-Inflammatory Orange Chicken and Spinach Salad	Anti-Inflammatory Salad	Black bean Buddha bowl with creamy cashew dressing	Deep Dish Falafel Pizza	Loaded sesame ginger salmon salad	Anti-Inflammatory Orange Chicken and Spinach Salad
Dinner	Lunch left-overs	Chicken and Snap Pea Stir-Fry	Yesterday's dinner left-overs	Lunch left-overs	Quick Orecchiette Pasta with Kale Pesto	Yesterday's dinner left-overs	Lunch left-overs

Anti-Inflammatory Diet

Week 2

	Sunday	Monday	Tuesday	Wednesday	Thursday	Friday	Saturday
Breakfast	Whole 30 Sweet Potato Protein Breakfast Bowl	Amaranth Porridge with Roasted Pears	Maple-baked rice porridge recipe with fruit	Turkey Apple Breakfast Hash (AIP)	Whole 30 Sweet Potato Protein Breakfast Bowl	Maple-baked rice porridge recipe with fruit	Amaranth Porridge with Roasted Pears
Lunch	Smoked salmon salad with green goddess dressing	Puttanesca-Style Beans and Greens	Loaded sesame ginger salmon salad	Black bean Buddha bowl with creamy cashew dressing	Anti-Inflammatory Salad	Yesterday's dinner left-overs	Yesterday's dinner left-overs
Dinner	Lunch left-overs	Curried red lentil and Swiss chard soup	Lunch left-overs	Lunch left-overs	Sweet Potato 'Rice' Casserole	White turkey chilli and avocado	Anti-Inflammatory Orange Chicken and Spinach Salad

Overcoming The Common Challenges, Fears And Uncertainties Concerning The Anti-Inflammatory Diet

Even with all we've discussed concerning what to eat and avoid, how to prepare your meals and how to plan, you will face certain challenges that will threaten your progress along the way and affect your ability to plan meals or going about the process itself.

Especially if you have children, a full-time job or busy schedules and many responsibilities, finding time to choose foods at the grocery store and make sure you prepare food on time and enjoy that food with people around you can be a challenge. That becomes worse when coupled with certain uncertainties and fears that most people have before they start.

I have addressed all possible challenges revolving around the anti-inflammatory diet to ensure you start with more confidence:

Challenge #1: Healthy meals take long to prepare!

Not always.

Always go for precut vegetables and other foods that are convenient to use like quartered marinated artichokes, pre-minced ginger and garlic, canned fish and beans, rotisserie-cooked chicken breasts, shredded cheese and the freshest produce (onions, broccoli, carrots, celery, cauliflower etc.) sold in the produce aisle to save time (this shortens the prep time and the ingredients last longer).

Challenge #2: What are the kids going to eat?

Most parents who are dieting make separate meals for their children. If you ask me, that's not always practical. Since good health is one of the best gifts you can give your kids, consider integrating them into the diet with these tips:

- *Customize the meal plan to suit your kids because they are different*

Kids sometimes wake up extremely famished and want a huge breakfast as soon as they open their eyes. Sometimes, they need some time to break a few things before their tummies start rumbling. How does your child wake up? This has to be reflected in your meal plan. Most children though, have to eat something every couple of hours, which means you have to prepare more food.

You also need to know the eating style of your kids and consider it while integrating them into the diet (if your kids are picky eaters, tweak your diet a bit more to include anti-inflammatory foods that are softer and crunchier and generally closer to what your kids like). However, you may have to incorporate more variety to make them less likely to oppose your new diet.

- *Make it a routine*

Kids are always open to trying out new things and a prudently-designed routine always works for them at the end of the day. They might not like the idea of not having to eat lots of sugary foods in the afternoon when you start making the changes, but with healthy food always showing up in the kitchen when they're hungry over and over again, eating the new foods will become a habit.

Challenge #3: how about eating out or ordering takeout?

We all know that it is not possible to cook 100% of our meals in advance, which means that there are times we have to eat at fast food joints and restaurants or order take-outs. Nonetheless, you can easily affect your progress negatively if you are not careful with the choices you make when eating out.

- *Take-outs*

You'll generally have to limit your takeout meals and eating out as much as possible because it's not very easy to find *true* anti-inflammatory meals from food outlets and restaurants.

Fast food is famous for its high fat, high sugar and high sodium content. But given that you already know what is expected of you when you start following an anti-inflammatory diet, I would not expect to see you rule fast food out completely.

All you need to do is ensure you order better than you've been doing. You can start by choosing restaurants that offer foods that are anti-inflammatory (or at least have a good record of delivering clean, whole, plant-based foods). Some good examples are In N Out and Carl's Jr. They can offer you grass fed, burgers and extra lettuce (in the place of the bun) among other meals consistent with the anti-inflammatory diet guidelines.

- *Restaurants*

At restaurants, it's easier to get what you want; when you make an order, you can ask for the right vegetable dressings and sauces to be brought along with it (you can also ask for extra servings). I will give you a few examples to ensure you always pull this off perfectly every time.

- <u>Italian food</u>

Italian food is not just about a large plate of pasta covered with cheese sauce; many restaurants provide many healthy Italian classics that you can take on an anti-inflammatory diet. A good example is Cioppino. This is a large bowl of fish stew, and is nearly the same as the French Bouillabaisse. These dishes are basically served with a classic tomato sauce and contain different types of seafood such as shrimp, mussels, clams and even fish.

When you decide to order this dish, don't forget to inform the waiter that you don't want a cream base, and also that you are dairy-intolerant (so that they bring something made without any dairy products) to ensure you avoid anything that is inflammatory.

When you want to eat lamb, you can also ask the waiter to get you extra vegetables to substitute anything inflammatory (like mashed potatoes or butter).

- Sushi

There are many reasons why you can eat sushi in restaurants without worrying that it might have inflammatory effects. I'm saying this because most people who are really ardent about healthy eating (or are generally strict with their dieting) fear sushi because of the rice. Lucky for us, we are currently living in an era where you can have a meal brought to you without a particular ingredient you don't want or like. There are definitely sushi rolls without rice but even if there weren't, you would still be able to order the food without the rice.

Sushi usually has many anti-inflammatory ingredients like ginger, seafood and vegetables which should be your main target ordering this kind of food. That also means you can ask for more vegetables on the side or ginger (for instance, you can ask for a nice spicy tuna with extra avocado and cucumber). Just ensure you avoid soy sauce because it is very inflammatory.

- Dessert

You already know how bad sugar is when it comes to inflammation but that doesn't mean you cannot enjoy desserts once in a while. Instead of selecting the ordinary desserts that are usually laden with sugar and dairy, go for ones that have been prepared with natural sweeteners like fruit. For instance, you can always ask for sugar-free sorbet.

Again, when it comes to great desserts, you can consider Thai food restaurants because they usually have coconut milk ice cream, dark chocolate covered strawberry and other great desserts that don't promote inflammation.

The bottom line is that you can decide to eat out and still enjoy the benefits of the anti-inflammatory diet and lifestyle just by ensuring you remember what you should eat and what you shouldn't and altering the way you order food. Indeed, you can eat many foods many people on a diet wouldn't dare touch just by making the appropriate requests.

Challenge #4: What happens if my meals start tasting bland?

This comes down to how dedicated you are to making this work. Most unhealthy foods are easy to prepare and don't require much effort to make them delicious. Healthy foods on the other hand require a bit more effort in terms of research and the process of preparation.

For instance, to make your diet work, you may have to stick a chart of spices/herbs and their matched foods inside your cupboard for reference to make better foods (for instance, with such a chart, you'll find new spices you probably didn't know about and the foods they best work with. I personally realized just the other day that thyme blends perfectly with chicken and mushrooms, and the fact that you can also use sundried tomatoes, balsamic vinegar and lemon juice to add some flavor to such a dish).

In other words, research for sustainable ways of making your food tastier.

Challenge 5: Healthy eating can be expensive!

Healthy eating is not always expensive. On the contrary, you can save a good amount of money substituting fresh veggies for all those different meat varieties, processed foods and salty snacks.

If you do the math, you'll realize that shopping at farmer markets or local food co-ops is a lot more cost effective than supermarkets. Trader Joe's and Whole Foods are actually offering lower pricing on most items!

Cooking your own food at home is another way to save cash. If you go out for lunch or dinner five days per week and spend $10 per meal, it means that you'll have used $26,000 by the end of the year! If you are usually too busy during the day, carrying your lunch to work is still an option.

Challenge 6: Giving up all my favorite foods is a big issue right now!

When you give yourself time and work on it every day, you'll be able to quit them.

The good thing is that the anti-inflammatory diet always encourages little, steady adjustments in what you eat. When you adopt the anti-inflammatory diet program, you start by increasing the amount and frequency of eating the good foods, and then replacing some of the pro-inflammatory foods with the anti-inflammatory foods step by step (for instance, eating a sweet fruit instead of a cookie) as you go.

If you used to eat cookies every day, you'll start eating more berries and less cookies progressively, and eventually replace the cookies with berries. When you replace most of the bad foods with good foods, make adjustments in the foods you store in the kitchen, and what you order or eat out and so on. Eventually, you should be able to cook completely different meals and eat completely different meals outside your house.

And in case you're worried about losing the pleasure of eating, you may want to note that even the folks diagnosed with chronic addiction eventually develop a taste for the healthy foods.

Obviously, you'll still crave your favorite unhealthy foods, and it is not bad to have them once in a while, but over time, you'll find yourself naturally choosing healthy foods without putting in too much effort. You'll find the anti-inflammatory diet even tastier when you begin seeing good results on yourself and feeling more energetic!

Challenge 7: I fear I might have a bad experience and fail like I did with the last diet.

In case you haven't noticed so far, the anti-inflammatory diet is not your typical diet (some people argue that it's not even a diet in the first place!).

First of all, people usually have bad experiences with diets because of their restrictive nature. Such diets only work for people who thrive under a lot of rules and regulations. It's difficult to have a bad experience with the anti-inflammatory diet because of its flexible nature; for instance, it doesn't have calorie limits, doesn't require apps to track anything, no cheat days and so on, yet it contains more benefits than most of those restrictive diets you'll see every day- including weight loss!

Indeed, the anti-inflammatory diet can assist you shed pounds in many ways. For instance, the foods keep you full for longer while keeping you energetic. Given that natural foods (which make up this diet) use a lot of energy to burn, your metabolism is always cranked up, and you get to burn more calories (to provide this energy) even when you are resting.

With such benefits and the ones we discussed earlier, it's nearly impossible to have a bad experience with this diet, if you do it right.

Enhance The Anti-Inflammatory Effects With Increased Physical Activity

Unfortunately, when most of us think of 'physical activity', what immediately comes to mind is a strict, regimented fitness routine- waking up at four in the morning to sweat until the sun comes to the rescue or going to the gym daily, for example. While I wouldn't dispute the fact that that's part of a healthy lifestyle, what matters first and foremost is what you do outside such strict routines, especially if you are looking to strengthen your immune system, lose weight and live a life free of inflammation in general.

Before you skip this part, my suggestion today is really simple:

1. *Sit less*

We all know that the average American adult sits for about 10 hours per day and the effects of this are too obvious to ignore. We are usually told that a one hour long workout at the end of the day can counteract this level of inactivity, but that's not true. You need to move almost continuously throughout the day- getting out of your chair every 45 minutes or so is a good place to start. Just to lay the groundwork for a great overall health, you should strive to sit for less than three hours per day, or get a stand-up desk if you really have to spend a lot of time at your desk.

2. Walk more

If you are really poor at determining what amounts to 'walking more', just get a good fitness tracker and use it to ensure you do about 7,000 to 10,000 steps per day. Of course, you can do more if you are enthusiastic enough, by not using your car in situations where you don't need it, taking nature walks and so on.

To make it even better, incorporate a convenient fitness routine.

3. Having a regimented workout

Many studies have been conducted in this area, and they have successfully shown the benefits of exercising when it comes to preventing and fighting inflammation; however, there's one particular study that really caught my attention titled

"The effects of intensive diet and exercises on knee joint loads, inflammation and clinical outcomes among overweight and obese adults with knee osteoarthritis."

https://www.ncbi.nlm.nih.gov/pubmed/24065013

This study clearly demonstrates how patients suffering from inflammation and pain improved more with a combination of exercise and dieting (compared to dieting or exercising alone). Therefore, while the anti-inflammatory diet is great for alleviating or preventing inflammation, combining it with good physical exercises can give you more than you expected. In this regard, I want you to do to things (apart from moving more):

✓ Engage in sports

Besides being one of the easiest programs on the list, it is also one of the most fun. All you have to do is play a sport you like, or even adopt a new sport and engage in it a couple of times each week. Since the idea is to get moving, some of the sports I'm thinking of right now are swimming, biking, football, rugby, rowing or padding and so forth. Sorry, darts, golf, chess and the like don't count.

When you choose your sport, begin with half an hour and progress gradually to 45 minutes and then 60 minutes per day, at least three days per week. If you can, try getting to 4-5 days per week.

✓ Engage in circuits

Basically, this entails doing one exercise, and another, followed by another one and so on until you complete a full circuit of exercises, then rest for a few minutes and repeat the entire circuit. The exercises can be cardio, strength exercises or a given combination. A circuit is great because it keeps things interesting and keeps your blood rushing, benefiting you more than exercises with long rests between the sets or exercises.

Of course, you'll have to start small- perhaps with 4-5 exercises and a resting period of 10-30 seconds between the exercises. With time, you can reduce the rest period until you get to a point where you can be able to complete the circuit without resting.

Which exercises should you do?

As a beginner, choose any four or five exercises such as jumping jacks, bodyweight squats, wall pushups, lunges, jogging, dips, burpees and jumping rope, depending on your level of fitness at the moment.

Arrange them based on a level of intensity and do 30 seconds of each, incorporating a 10-30 seconds rest between them. When you complete all four or five, take a two-minute rest and repeat.

When you're just starting, stick to 2 circuits and then add a third circuit after one or two weeks. In your fourth week, you should be able to at least four circuits. When you become fully adjusted to the wonderful life of working out, you will find yourself adding more and more exercises, and switching exercises all the time.

Conclusion

We have come to the end of the book. Thank you for reading and congratulations for reading until the end.

If you are happy with the book, can you please leave a review?

www.ingramcontent.com/pod-product-compliance
Lightning Source LLC
Chambersburg PA
CBHW030157100526
44592CB00009B/329